DIRTY TALK BIBLE

How Men and Women Can Have Mind-Blowing Sexual Experiences Simply by "Talking Dirty" (2022 Guide for Beginners)

Kenelm Little

TABLE OF CONTENTS

INTRODUCTION

It's easy to talk. At least, that's what we've been taught. We've been programmed to believe that when it comes to sex, it all comes down to action. The most experienced lovers, on the other hand, understand that a single word can have the power of a thousand caresses.

Magnolia refers to the discussion of sexually charged topics. It is the act of increasing pleasure before and during a sexual act by using vivid word imagery. However, contrary to popular belief, dirty talking does not always have to be an outpouring of the filthiest, most derogatory phrases. Unless, of course, the latter piques your interest. Simply put, there are no specific definitions, rules, or boundaries when it comes to dirty talk. Its beauty stems from its lack of boundaries.

The lexicon of lust may include derogatory words, reverent words, or no words at all. Dirty talk can range from a sigh to a single syllable to a torrent of hot obscenities. It's a poet's intense erotic descriptions, a dominant's powerful command, a submissive's vow of obedience, and the guttural growl of a lover blinded by animal lust. Furthermore, dirty talk does not always have to be said. It can be whispered into the ear of a lover, spoken over the phone, or scribbled as a short, sexy note.

While dirty talk has long been used as a form of foreplay, it can also occur during or after intercourse. What you say before, during, and after the act is equally important. A single hot word can send your lover to a mind-blowing climax, but it can also be used to caress his or her delicate ego as he or she descends from the peak. Dirty talk, when used after lovemaking, can have the effect of the sweetest cuddle or a shower of grateful kisses. This means that dirty talk is more than just a way to arouse lust. It is also one of the most daring and, ironically, one of the warmest and tender expressions of love and affection. Dirty talk, when used to boost your lover's confidence in bed, can bring out his or her most free, passionate side. Apart from inevitably improving the quality of your lovemaking, it has the potential to transform sex from a primal act of pleasure to an enlightening journey of self-discovery.

The language of lust, like sex, is subjective. What may irritate some may drive others insane with desire. It is for this reason that simply memorizing a list of strange words is insufficient. Knowing when and how to say things is just as important as knowing what to say.

The expression in your eyes, the tone of your voice, your facial expression, and your body posture are all important in shaping the meaning behind each word. All of these factors, along with the context, influence how your partner perceives and responds to your steamy expressions. All of these factors work together to determine the sincerity and weight of passion contained in your verbal declarations of desire. Dirty talking is, without a doubt, an art form. It is necessary to study and practice to be effective. Fortunately for you, this is the subject of this book.

So, are you ready to learn the language of desire? Continue reading to find out how.

CHAPTER 1:

THE PSYCHOLOGY BEHIND THE LANGUAGE OF LUST

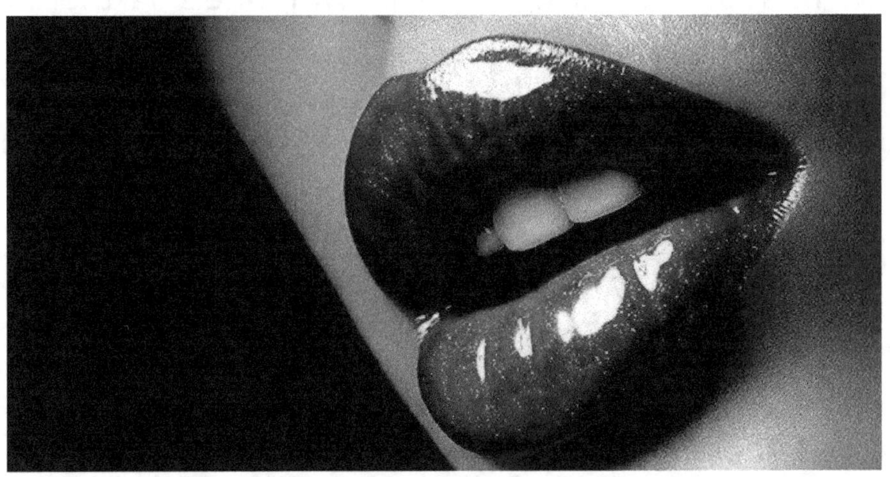

Perhaps the most appealing aspect of dirty talk is the fact that it is still considered taboo. You're probably thinking to yourself, "Taboo?" You're joking! We are living in enlightened times... Even though we have emerged from the Dark Ages, the reality is that sex is still frowned upon. The human mind has been pre-programmed to perceive sex as a delicate act that is only performed and discussed behind closed doors.

We're not going to be able to get rid of this easily. So, despite our liberated front and over-sexed culture, despite the availability of pornographic materials, even talking or reading about sex can cause a tingle of excitement or stir a secret shame within.

Our parents have taught us since we were children that saying bad words is, well, bad. But now that we're adults, breaking that rule with one's partner in bed feels oh-so-good.

It's akin to saying, "Fuck yes! I'm a grown man/woman, and I'm in charge. Nobody is going to stop me or shame me for saying whatever I want." Unfortunately, not all adults are as liberated. Some people are still subconsciously bound by old rules. As a result, even in bed, they strive to be good girls and boys. That's not to say they're immature. Rather, the shackles of societal conventions may bind them too tightly. But that's all part of the appeal of dirty talk! The fact that you can say what you can't say in front of others makes lovemaking more intimate, rawer, and real. When that bedroom door closes and the first vile word escapes your lips, that's when you strip naked in front of your lover.

In some ways, speaking out about all the weird things that are going through your head is more revealing than taking your clothes off. After all, you only expose your body in the latter, whereas you expose your soul in the former.

Sex is created in the brain first. 80 per cent of the sex we have in our lives takes place in our heads. These include carnal memories, desire buildup, and conscious and subconscious fantasies. These are the motivating factors that influence everything we do during the actual intimate act. Your brain has been building up to the erotic encounter by the time you slip into the sheets. In other words, even before you start getting physical with your lover, your mind has fondled and fucked him/her a thousand times.

Perhaps you've heard that the brain is the largest and most powerful sex organ that men and women share.

After all, the brain contains an infinite supply of sensual stimuli, and it is from here that the sex drive emerges. When you moan, scream, or whisper something into your lover's ear, the hearing centre of his or her brain processes it. The temporal, frontal, and occipital lobes also process it. So, while this vital sexual organ is not physically touched, dirty talk before and during sex allows you to lick, caress, and fuck various parts of your lover's brain all at once, all while pleasing your partner's body.

Dirty words are the quickest and most certain way to fuck your lover's brains out.

True, the right amount and type of carnal conversation can titillate your lover's mind. Yes, you read that correctly. There is such a thing as the right kind and amount of dirty talk. This is because men's and women's brains are wired differently. There is a significant difference in how male and female limbic systems function in the brain.

According to scientific evidence, the preoptic area, or the section of the hypothalamus responsible for mating behaviour, is twice as large in males as it is in females. Furthermore, it has twice as many cells. In other words, men have a larger hypothalamus. So, what does all of this mean? Because gonadotropin-releasing hormone from the hypothalamus stimulates testosterone production, men have higher levels of circulating male sex hormone. This, in turn, increases their desire for sex. In contrast, in the case of the female, which has a smaller hypothalamus, testosterone, and thus sex drive, is not nearly as high.

Women associate romance with emotions, whereas men associate romance with sexual affirmation. While sex for a man is about affirming his vitality and manhood, sex for a woman is about being reassured that she is attractive, accepted, and adored. As a result, if you're a woman, using dirty words that praise your manhood is a surefire way to pique your man's interest. Simply put, you worship him if you worship his cock. If you're a man, complimenting your woman's body is a surefire way to get her in the mood for love. In other words, if you make her feel like a goddess, she will act like a goddess in bed.

Dirty talk works by providing your partner with exactly what he or she requires.

According to studies, many women who hold dominant positions in their careers prefer to play a more submissive role on the sheets. In the workplace, the woman may be the boss. She could be the one issuing all the orders. But, to get excited in bed, she needs to feel something she doesn't get to feel in her everyday life: vulnerability. When you command her in a dominant tone, the amygdala, or fear centre of her brain, is stimulated. This takes control away from her, which is what makes it exciting for her. More importantly, you're relieving her of the burden of responsibility. This enables her to simply let go. Because, for once, it is not her responsibility to be in charge of everything.

In the heat of passion, it's easy to lose sight of what the other person is feeling. This is why many lovers make the mistake of ignoring their partner's needs during a critical stage of lovemaking. Dirty conversation during sex allows us to be more open to our partner's immediate needs and desires, allowing us to meet those needs. To put it another way, dirty talk enables us to become more sensitive, generous lovers.

At the same time, dirty talking during sex allows us to express our desires and wants without sounding too selfish or demanding.

Many self-help books on the subject of sex will advise you to keep lines of communication open in bed. They will tell you to be truthful, informative, and respectful. This way, you and your partner can both get what you want and need from each other. What they don't mention is that there is an art to it.

Some sex manuals will tell you to simply zip it.

They will advise you to keep talking to a minimum during intercourse because it can distract your lover and possibly ruin the mood.

Which of these books, then, is preaching the truth? Here's a little known fact:

Both are correct. While feedback is essential for great sex, any words that come out of your mouth can divert your and your lover's attention away from the moment. Furthermore, any words spoken during sex can easily be misconstrued.

Consider the following example:

"Please don't come before I do, Honey."

To put it politely? Yes.

Honest? Surely.

Instructive? Definitely.

Sexy? No, not quite.

Distracting? Very.

Such a statement could make your lover look bad. So, rather than being helpful and improving the quality of lovemaking, you end up making your partner feel selfish, inadequate, or that his lovemaking style stinks. Furthermore, such a statement will only reveal that you are nowhere near achieving orgasm. While this is true, it is not something your lover should hear while he is figuratively (and literally) busting his balls trying to get you to come with him.

While some may consider dirty talk to be offensive, it is, in fact, the most non-offensive way of communicating your wants and needs to your partner. Just look at the "falsified" version below:

"Oooh... That feels fantastic, hon. Keep doing that, and I'll come at you hard!"

See? The thing about dirty talk is that it always goes hand in hand with your dirty deed. As a result, you can instruct without being distracted. It allows you to be honest about the fact that you're not yet at climax without making your lover feel like a loser. Instead, it motivates your partner to work harder so that he or she can reap the incomparably satisfying reward of making you come... so hard.

Dirty talk allows you and your partner to be honest with each other and get to know each other in the most intimate way possible.

There is constant pressure in everyday life to conform to society's standards. You are only allowed to say certain things. There are only a few options available to you. Dirty talk allows you and your lover to connect with your more primal, creative sides. In other words, it awakens the animal within, without fear, shame, or guilt. This refers to the wild and sensual side of ourselves that is frequently lost, forgotten, and allowed to wither and die. This part is frequently suppressed by our fear of being judged, being labelled a freak, or losing the love of our partner. However, lovemaking will never be as fulfilling until both of your inner beasts can face and embrace each other without anxiety or embarrassment. Only when you and your partner can see through each other and accept what you see within each other can you truly call yourselves intimate lovers. Only then can you truly call someone your soulmate?

You are free to stand naked in front of anyone. You can kiss, caress, and make love to anyone. But to allow someone to read your mind when you're at your most vulnerable? This necessitates trust. This necessitates a special kind of love.

If you're not sure if your partner is ready for your idea of fun, some dirty talking is a great way to test the waters. Consider it lube to smooth the way before fucking your lover in ways he/she has never imagined being fucked before. For example, if your bedmate still cringes when called a slut, he or she is probably not ready to be treated as one. If, on the other hand, your lover appears to respond positively to the word, chances are he or she is open to the idea. And we've all seen how easily words can turn into actions.

Naughty lingo stimulates the senses. That is the creative juices.

As previously stated, 80 per cent of sexual activity occurs within the brain.

When words are spoken aloud, they have a way of becoming ingrained in the subconscious. As a result, if you tell your lover what you intend to do to him/her, the erotic scenario will replay in your mind until the opportunity to get physical arises.

At this point, the scenario will no longer be a fantasy.

For example, if a man tells his woman, "I'm going to fuck you on your desk and show you who's boss," the image of his woman bent over her desk, skirt hiked up, and panties around her ankles will be tattooed on his brain until it becomes unbearably vivid. He'll come up with ideas for how to make this fantasy a reality. He'll pay her a surprise visit in her office soon.

Some sexual fantasies may be difficult for us to turn into reality. Perhaps we aren't quite ready yet.

Maybe we'll never be prepared for them. Nonetheless, dirty talk can serve as a springboard to fulfilling those fantasies. If not, it can at least allow us to live out some of our fantasies. While you may not want to beat the snot out of your wife or husband, playing with harsh words (ex: Stay down or I'll slap you, you filthy whore.) can be a satisfying and even therapeutic alternative.

You're probably thinking, "Why?" Why would a woman (or man) who is naturally offended by the term "whore" outside the bedroom be fine with it during sex? The answer is straightforward:

When the term "whore" or "slut" is used outside of the bedroom, it takes on the meaning that society has given it. That is, a person with shaky morals who allows anyone and everyone to escape from his or her body. When used privately in bed, however, the woman/man has complete control over the world, giving it its definition.

He or she can use it on his or her terms. A "whore" could be someone who is extremely flexible in bed or someone who has a body that is so hot that there is no decent word for it. A "slut" is someone who consumes cum. Or maybe not. It could be someone who allows his or her partner to fuck him or her up the a$$. Or maybe not. "Whore" does not have to imply "cheap." "Slut" does not have to be impure. Unless, of course, you want it to be.

Dirty talk allows you to connect.

It ensures that you and your lover are on the same wavelength.

Screams of pleasure are always welcome, but the problem is that they are easily misinterpreted. One particularly aggravating, yet surprisingly common, scenario is when your partner stops doing something delightful because he or she misinterprets your moans of pleasure for moans of pain. There's no better way to put a stop to a sexy mood. Situations like these are easily avoidable if only one dares to speak up and say what is on one's mind. "Oh, baby, don't you dare stop!" is a simple way to tell your lover that he or she is on the right track.

Dirty talk is all about stroking the ego. The language of lust is about encouraging one another.

The majority of people will agree that sex is more than just a physical release. It is an expression of affection. It's a form of emotional bonding. More than that, it is a healing act. When done correctly, lovemaking can assist lovers in processing major and minor traumas together. We help each other's sense of self-worth by having sex. We support one another's development. Your words have the power to transform a timid flower into a voluptuous goddess. Your words have the power to make a man feel unbreakable. Women, in particular, are self-conscious about their bodies. Despite appearances, men are constantly concerned about their sexual performance. "God, your breasts are beautiful!" or "I love the way your cock fills me up." is a miraculous elixir against all the insecurities that have held your partner down for the majority of his/her life.

Dirty talk is an expression of appreciation and gratitude at the end of lovemaking.

"I didn't just fuck you," naughty words can mean. It was fantastic." It's also a way of saying, "I didn't just fuck you." "I adore you." in a completely non-awkward tone. It makes no difference whether your goal is to express your feelings or to secure a second invitation into a lover's bed. If you use dirty talk to boost your lover's confidence genuinely, he or she will want to sleep with you again and again. By complimenting your lover's efforts with filthy phrases such as "God, I love coming deep in your throat." or

"My pussy is still raw from riding your cock... I'd do it again in a heartbeat.", you are adding emotional gratification to their physical satisfaction. In the end, you'll be the best, most thorough lover he or she has ever had.

CHAPTER 2:

BUILDING YOUR CARNAL CONFIDENCE

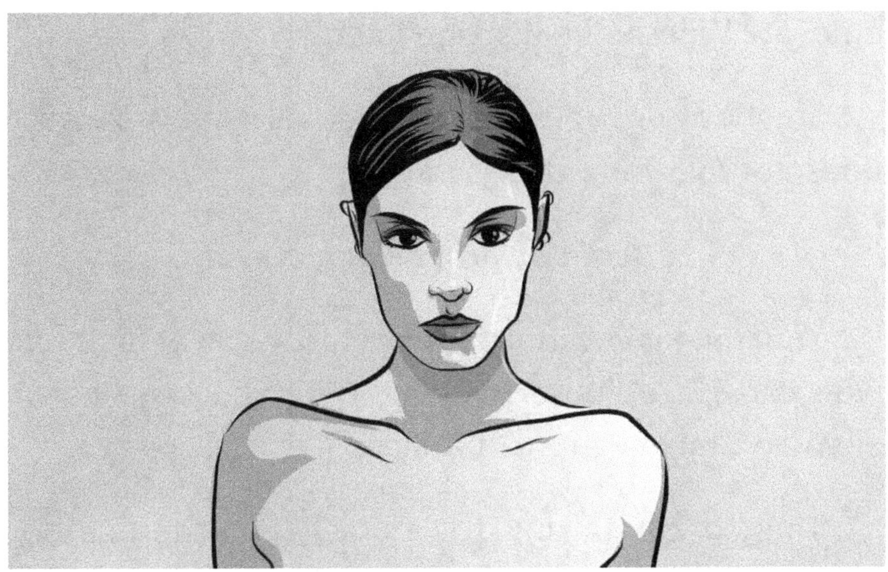

Speaking is supposed to be simple. You've been doing it since you were a child, after all. But why is dirty talking so difficult? The truth is that even the most talkative people and the most imaginative writers find playful pillow talk difficult. Some words that appear erotic in print may sound downright embarrassing when spoken aloud. Even the most sexually confident men and women will come across a naughty word that will cause them to blush from head to toe. This is because, historically, sex has always been about the act.

Dirty talking made you feel as if you were stripping your clothes off over and over again at first. With each word, a new layer peels away, and you wait with bated breath to see how your partner reacts. Will he enjoy it? Will she be disconnected?

So, how do you ensure that all that sexy talk doesn't drive your lover away?

Begin by practising yourself.

Your vulgar vocabulary may startle you at first, but who cares? You'll be the only one who can hear it anyway. Start by masturbating.

Then begin talking to yourself in a derogatory manner. You don't need to have a large vocabulary at this point. Simply use simple words. Concentrate on the pleasure and think aloud. Staying silent is a hundred times hotter than blurting out an honest sentence like, "Oh yeah, that feels good."

After that, imagine you're having sex with your lover. In any case, it's what you do when you masturbate. If you're a guy, imagine your cock in her pussy as you slip your cock into your lubed-up fist. So, rather than saying, "Oh yeah, that feels good," say, "Oh yeah, your pussy feels good."

Imagine his cock as you slide your fingers in and out of you if you're a woman. So, rather than saying, "Oh yeah, that feels good," say, "Oh yeah, your cock feels so good."

Nonetheless, words like "good" are far too broad. When it comes to sexy talk, the more specific you are, the more impact you will have. Describe your feelings in your head as you continue to imagine yourself making love to your partner. Adjectives can help to bring those sensations to life.

"Oh my gosh, your pussy is so fucking tight!"

"Oh, your cock is fucking thick!"

However, anyone's cock can be thick. Anyone's pussy can be constrictive. The dirty talk must hit home to be effective. Furthermore, when using adjectives, you must exercise caution and stick as closely to the truth as possible. For example, don't call a man's cock "thick" when you both know it isn't.

As a result, the next step is to consider your partner. What's his/her personality like? What do you think he/she would most like to hear? What do you believe he or she needs to hear the most?

Is he constantly concerned about his weight? "Baby, I love how your cock fits me perfectly," you could say.

Is she self-conscious about her voluminous boobs? Tell her how it feels like heaven to bury your face in them.

You're getting pretty good at this, don't you? Masturbate and practice your dirty talk with a tape recorder as you become more comfortable and talkative. This way, you'll know whether you need to talk more or less, whether you need to speak louder or softer, or whether you need to dial back the naughtiness a notch.

Develop a positive attitude and keep an open mind.

Most people's qualms stem from the belief that dirty talk somehow devalues them, their partners, or their relationships. To become erotically eloquent, you must dispel the myth that using dirty words makes sex unclean. One thing to remember is that a person's sexual persona is only one aspect of himself/herself. Your lover is not just who he or she is in the sack. It does not reflect who he or she is outside of the bedroom. Your genital organs are not filthy.

The genitals of your partner are not filthy. By using simple words to refer to them (for example, cunt, penis, pussy, cock, breasts, boobs, vagina, balls, etc.), you are asserting that these body parts are not to be ashamed of, but rather deserve to be appreciated and thus mentioned.

Try out the following activity:

In front of a mirror, stand naked. Examine and touch your genitals. Take note of them. Determine and describe your favourite aspects of them.

For example, my breasts are a real handful. My nipples are small and attractive. I adore their sensitivity!

or

My breasts are large and full. I enjoy playing with them because they are soft and bouncy.

Make an effort to focus on the positive aspects of your life. And never, ever compare yourself to the airbrushed vaginas and surgically enhanced penises seen in pornographic movies and magazines. Ex: If you're conscious of how your labia minora is an outie, consider how awesome it is that your guy gets to nibble on some flesh during cunnilingus.

Discuss sex with your partner. It's the right thing to do.

The more at ease you are discussing sex with your lover, the easier it will be to transition to dirty talk. After you've had sex, get close to your partner and tell him or her how you felt.

Mention your favourite bedroom tricks and lovemaking positions. Tell your lover what you want her/him to do over and over.

Ex: When you put a vibrator on my clit while you went down on me, I went insane. I can't wait until you do it again.

Make your points clear. Make a graphic. It was hot when your lover did it to you, but hearing the act described through your lips will make it even hotter. Take note of your lover's reaction. His/her reaction will give you an idea of how he/she feels about smutty speech.

Never, ever pass judgment.

The bed should be a haven from the outside world. Just as you don't criticize your partner when he or she shows you his or her body, don't criticize your lover when he or she bears his or her thoughts.

Recognize that speaking openly necessitates trust. Being vocal before, during, or after intercourse increases one's vulnerability. As a result, resist the urge to laugh or react angrily during a sexy conversation. Don't chastise your lover for using inappropriate words during sex or foreplay. Discuss it at least a few hours later.

Ex: Remember when we were having fun and you referred to me as a cum dumpster? That was a little too filthy for me."

Dirty talk does not permit you to be disrespectful.

Create a set of rules with your partner to prevent dirty talk from becoming too dirty for your tastes. Discuss which words you are and are not comfortable with.

"I'm fine with being called a gutter whore," for example. Just don't refer to me as a bang hole."

It's all about giving and taking when it comes to great lovemaking. It's simple for the more talkative partner to dominate the dirty talk. However, consider dirty talking to be an opportunity for the more silent person to verbalize more. It's one way to get to know your lover better. When acting out roles, remember to take turns and to always be on the same page. If one is a slave, the other has to be the master. There can never be two masters at the same time. Furthermore, being able to put yourself in the shoes of both the listener and the speaker will allow you to form a reasonable perspective.

"Come on, honey, let's do the chocolate cha."

Does the term "anal sex" conjure up images of feces? If it does, you are not required to use it in your coital conversations. Feel free to invent your lust lingo that you'll be able to understand.

Remember, the goal of dirty talk is to arouse you, not to disgust you. Making your secret dirty dialect will also serve to deepen your intimacy with your lover.

Don't make the mistake of going with the same old, same old stuff once you've worked up the courage to talk dirty.

Avoid using the same phrases over and over. For God's sake, you've come so far; don't squander it! Make an effort to be unpredictable. After all, dirty talk is ten times more effective when you catch your partner off guard. Experiment with various voices and step outside of your comfort zone. Be a Casanova one moment and a caveman the next.

When it comes to mastering steamy bedroom talk, expanding your lewd vocabulary is a valuable tool. For some, the penis and vagina may appear overly clinical. Experiment with different terms instead of saying pussy or the commonly used cunt. (honeysuckle, juice box, Altar of Venus, and so forth) Similarly, numerous words can be substituted for cock (joystick, cum gun, fuck rod, etc.). Consider your feelings about incorporating these words into your lovemaking routine.

Are they too obnoxious? Is it too clean? Is it too medical? Too obnoxious? Make a list of modern sex jargon and read it with your partner.

Choose the ones you think are hot. Laugh at the amusing ones. The corny ones will make you roll your eyes. Make it enjoyable!

How many times can the words "great," "hot," and "good" be used before they become stale? Increase your knowledge of carnal adjectives.

Make a list of words to describe your partner's vagina. Wet, slick, and warm are fine, but how about luscious, plump, succulent, and lip-smacking? Similarly, while hard and long are good, the words iron, enormous, and powerful can also be used to describe a dick.

The same is true when you describe your lovemaking and climaxes. Saying "That was amazing." sounds great the first, second, and possibly even third time, but by the fourth time, the compliment is likely to sound more mechanical and less genuine. To describe a satisfying orgasm, use words like earth-shattering, out-of-this-world, and spine-tingling.

CHAPTER 3:

FILTHY FLIRTING

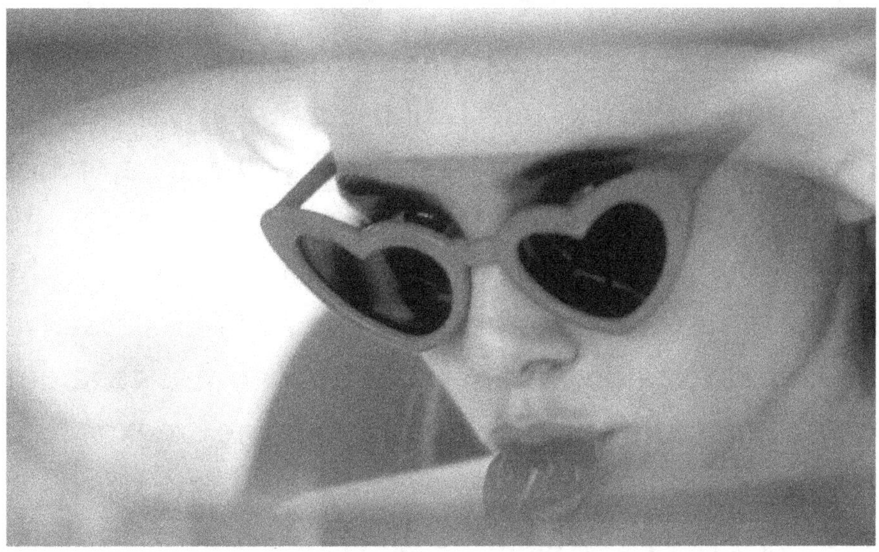

When flirting, using dirty talk can help spice up an existing relationship and keep it from becoming stale. Similarly, you can use some naughty talk to set the tone for a new relationship. This is especially useful when meeting new people. In this case, your goal is to keep yourself from falling into the friend zone.

Tips and Tricks for Dirty Seduction for Men

Girls, on the other hand, tend to like to play hard to get. This isn't always a bad thing. Men, after all, were created to enjoy the thrill of the hunt. In other words, when it comes to sex, a large part of the thrill is in the ride leading up to the moment when he finally finds himself deep inside his conquest.

Seducing a girl is simple if she believes you're a great guy. The tricky part is figuring out how to appear nice without appearing so nice that you end up on her list of unfuckable guy pals. Some might argue that the most obvious solution would be to hit on her right away. Demonstrate to her that you find her attractive and want to sleep with her. But how do you go about doing this without offending her? The unexpected response would be to have her do all of the work for you. Yes, you should be the one to start the dirty talk. However, do it in such a way that she believes it was all her idea.

If you're a guy, here are a few tried-and-true things you can say to a girl to make her see you as the man she'll inevitably have sex with, not just any man.

Inquire as to what she puts on before going to bed.

What is the procedure for this? It causes her to consider the bed. This seemingly innocuous question is enough to spark a discussion about sexy lingerie and intimate bedtime rituals. Take note of her reaction. If the question makes her feel uncomfortable, back off a little. She's not interested in talking about her nighttime routine with you. When a girl starts talking about her cute pyjamas, panties, or nightgown, that's your cue to move on.

Continue to: **Do you enjoy sleeping naked?**

This will cause her to consider nudity and her body. And, of course, there's sex.

Inquire about her most fashionable outfit.

It all sounds so innocent, but it will give you an idea of what she considers sexy. This works not only with new acquaintances but also with long-term lovers. You might be surprised at how much you can learn about your girlfriend's or wife's secret sexual fantasies by asking her what she considers to be the most provocative number in her wardrobe. Hopefully, your long-term lover is just waiting for the right moment to show you her spankin' hot costume.

Inquire if she has ever observed another couple having fun.

It's not like you're inquiring about her sexual life. You're inquiring about the sexual activities of others. As a result, she is likely to feel more at ease. She'll get your point and join in if she wants to. You'll know if she doesn't want to take you any further.

After all, it's simple for her to deny witnessing another couple commit the heinous crime. On the other hand, if she's up for it, she'll go into great detail about the erotic encounter. This allows you to move on to more questions with sensual undertones. As an example...

Have you ever kissed a guy simply because you were hot and bothered?

This question will show her that you're not one of those guys who thinks of women as the less sexual gender. Ladies experience strong and unexpected bursts of lust, and they act on these impulses without shame or guilt. This question will give your date a chance to show you her wild side. More than that, it's one way of signalling to her that you're down if she wants to jump you and have a good time right now.

Pose a hypothetical question to your date that focuses her attention on the male anatomy.

"Assume you're going on a blind date." Almost blind. Assume you'll have the opportunity to examine one part of the man's body. His face isn't included in this. "Which part of your body would you like to see?"

Unless she's a complete prude, there's no way she'd refuse to answer this question. After all, you're not talking about your naked body. Nonetheless, she will unavoidably think about you and your body as a result of this. Furthermore, this allows you to determine which part of the male anatomy she thinks is the sexiest.

Encourage her to discuss why she chose this body part if she responds positively to this question. Why does she like it so much? What if it piques her interest?

Then, get her to think about your body.

Ask her a casual and somewhat silly question, such as, "Do you think I'll look better with or without more body hair?"

While it's unlikely that this question will spark a deeper conversation, you've succeeded in getting her to imagine you naked, so you've done your job.

As the conversation progresses, inquire playfully about any secret moves she employs to entice men.

Encourage her to elaborate on her response. This conversation topic can be used in both directions. Her response may turn you on, but the more she talks about it and thinks about it, the more it makes her feel frisky.

When she goes into detail about her special sexual moves, you'll know she's into the dirty talk.

If you and your lady have been dating for a while, ask her questions like, "Of all the sexy things you've done to me, which one was your favourite?"

Which sex position would you prefer if we could only make love in one?

This question may lead to further investigation, such as why this sex pose feels so good or why it makes her come harder than any other position. She'll end up talking about how this or that position makes your cock feel incredibly large or how it allows your penis to hit her in all the right places.

Inquire about the specific part of her body that puts her in the mood for love.

The answer will provide you with information about your date's preferences in the sheets. More importantly, this steamy question will cause her to conjure up a vivid mental image. The more she describes her erogenous zones, the more she'll think about them and become aroused.

Start the dirty talk with questions like these if you're flirting with a long-term lover:

What does it feel like when I touch you?

Do you mind if I lick you?

What part of your body would you like me to kiss more frequently?

The next step is to get her to fantasize about having sex with you.

Ask her a question like, "If there's anything I can do to turn you on, what would it be?"

This will demonstrate to her that you genuinely care about what she enjoys in bed and strive to please her.

Hold your girlfriend or wife close or look into her eyes and ask racy questions like, *"How can I make you wetter than you've ever been?"*

What can I do to entice you to return?

Remind her of all the hot things you've done to get her to imagine having sex with you.

Ex: *Do you remember when we had our first kiss on the beach? We were all sweating profusely. Your pussy tasted deliciously sweet and salty. I can't seem to get it out of my head.*

You can keep asking naughtier, more direct questions as the lust-filled back and forth continues.

For example, how do you feel about oral sex?

Have you ever made love in front of others?

What is the most daring sex position you've ever tried?

Have you ever used a sex toy? What did you think of it?

How do you feel about masturbation? How frequently do you do it?

Have you ever gotten wet while getting a massage?

Continue to gauge her reactions as you do so. Curt's replies indicate that it is time to move on to a more civilized topic. Answers that are detailed indicate that it is safe to proceed.

If you think you need to calm down, talk about something nonsexual before turning the heat back up with more teasing questions.

These are gentler conversation starters, but they have the potential to heat things depending on how far the lady wants to take it:

What is the naughtiest, sexiest movie or work of literature you've ever seen/read? Did it pique your interest?

What is the naughtiest/sexiest thing you've ever done?

Have you ever skinny dipped?

What are your feelings about sexting?

Assuming everything goes as planned and she's completely open to your titillating talk, it's time to ask the game-changers, the questions that will turn words into actions.

Is this conversation turning you on?

If that's the case, tell her what you intend to do to her. (For example, This conversation makes me want to slide my hand up your skirt and feel you.)

What would you say if I touched you now?

Could I kiss you?

In their simplicity, these statements are powerful. This shows her how much you adore her. If she gives you the go-ahead for a kiss, go ahead and do it.

If you've been having sex with a woman for a long time, keep the fire burning by asking risqué questions in public:

Ex: While dining out, say something to her like this: *"How would you feel if I ran my hand up your skirt and slipped a finger inside you?"*

The great thing about her smart, strategic approach is that she'll be doing the majority of the dirty talking. You won't have to repeatedly and nervously dip your toe in the water, nor will you have to constantly worry about offending her with each word. You're allowing your lady to reveal as much or as little as she wants by asking these provocative questions. In other words, she has control over the level of filthiness in dirty talk. You'll make her feel like she's a bad, bad girl in her own right. You are, in a sense, empowering her. That sense of power will be extremely attractive to her.

Women's Dirty Seduction Tips and Tricks

You vs. The Good Girl

The Good Girl Complex is one of the most difficult obstacles for women to overcome when learning how to talk dirty. Girls grow up aspiring to be the ultimate good girl in their quest for affirmation from others. They work hard to get good grades, and then they excel at work.

They go out of their way to please others to be labelled "beautiful" or "perfect." This complex affects even ostensibly "bad" girls. While they may engage in self-destructive behaviours, the result is the same: they will still bend over backwards to gain the attention or acceptance of others. This need to feel "good enough" for others, this strong desire to be valued, leads women to ignore their own inner needs and desires. It deafens them to their voice. They become strangers to their sexual persona as a result. It is for this reason that so many women are pushed to engage in sexual acts before they are sure they are ready.

Following that, they feel guilty and "atone" for their actions by resuming the good girl image.

Proper women (aka the women worth bringing home to Ma) were traditionally expected to be pure and innocent. However, we all know that a lady on the street is not every man's dream come true, but a whore in the sheets! If you're a woman, you have to stop worrying about what your man will think of you once you utter that first naughty phrase. Perhaps you're concerned that he'll think you're slutty.

That's fine. The trick is to convince him that you are not a slut, but that you can be one for him.

According to research, women are less likely to initiate the dirty talk. Make the first move if you want to. Breaking free from the good girl mould can be liberating and empowering. If you're afraid of being rejected, start with vague phrases that may or may not be sexual.

Ex: **I'll tell you about it later. *You're going to enjoy it a lot.***

Of course, the key to injecting a hint of sensuality into statements like these is to use your voice, facial expressions, and body language.

Look him in the eyes if you want to add a touch of sexiness to this statement. In a casual tone, say the first sentence.

Then, lean in close and whisper something into his ear. For the second sentence, lower your voice. Make it a little huskier. Pull back and finish with a small, amusing smile. Then you should leave.

Lean in closer and show him your cleavage if you want it to be extra sexy. Allow your breasts to lightly brush against his upper arm as you whisper in his ear.

Keep in mind that men are visual beings. This section will show you how different dirty talk techniques are for men and women.

Other sexy but seemingly innocent conversation starters that could lead to raunchy talk include:

Do you think you could beat me in an arm wrestle if I challenged you?

I'm going to need you to tell me something... What's the big deal about threesomes?

Which do you prefer: boobs or butts?

I was thinking about going celibate for about two years. What are your thoughts?

What if I told you that I have a secret twin sister who looks exactly like me?

Who would you choose to sleep with if you could only sleep with one celebrity?

Choose one: I'm going to live the rest of my life in sweatpants. Or I wear short, tight black dresses for the rest of my life.

Here are some more direct dirty conversation starters for men who like it:

Have you ever had a neighbour complain about how loud you were in bed?

Tell me about your favourite wild thing you've done during sex.

What's your most racy, X-rated sexual fantasy?

What is the most heinous, sexiest thing you've ever done to someone?

Which part of your body do you think is the sexiest? What would you do if I got your hands on it?

Have you ever been caught masturbating in public?

If you've been sleeping with a guy for a while, try these suggestions:

What would you say if you caught me having sex with a supermodel?

Last night, I had a dream about you. I awoke drenched.

Last night, I couldn't sleep. I needed you by my side.

Have you ever dreamed about me? What were we up to?

Guess the colour of the pants I'm wearing. Assuming I'm wearing one, of course...

When was the last time you brushed up against yourself? Please tell me about it.

The sentences that follow are not guaranteed to spark further discussion. These are powerful bombs that you simply drop before leaving or switching to another topic. Just make sure to use phrases like these sparingly. They work best when you catch the guy off guard.

I'm not sure... Something about you makes me feel so... feminine.

You have this thing you do. It's fantastic. But I can't tell you. Because if I do, you'll stop doing it.

I like the cologne you're wearing. It's very... masculine.

Caressing a man's ego and dirty talking will do you wonders.

When teasing a guy, especially in the early stages of a relationship, keep the dirty talk light and playful. This way, if he's not into it, you can easily save face and continue talking about something else.

Talking Dirty to Your Long-Term Partner

Boredom is a harbinger of the end of any relationship. It may appear unfair, but women in long-term relationships are constantly striving to keep things interesting and fun for their men, lest they seek entertainment elsewhere. They can't help themselves. As previously stated, they were hardwired to crave the hunt. Talking dirty is one way to keep the excitement in your relationship going. That doesn't mean you should start saying things that would make a pornstar blush. As previously stated, it is simple to arouse your man by saying completely non-sexual things.

Ex: *I like how you wear those jeans.*

That's right, ladies: men, too, deserve to be complimented! For married couples who have been together for a long time: When was the last time, you told your husband how much you adore his a$$? Or how about that sexy dream you had about him?

The preceding example is effective because it draws attention to the man's genital zone.

To avoid boredom, alternate between soft-core and hard-core dirty talk.

Soft-core dirty talk phrases: I desperately need you.

When you look at me like that, it makes me happy.

That thing you do with your tongue... It drives me insane.

The key to making soft-core dirty talk work is to say it correctly.

The great thing about these seemingly innocent phrases is that they can go from mildly naughty to extremely wicked with a simple change in tone of voice, gaze direction, or context. Take a look at the following example:

"You're unbelievably hot."

If you say this to his face while looking him in the eyes, it sounds like a flattering compliment. But what if you say the same thing with gritted teeth, a gruff voice, and while grabbing his biceps? The words sound hotter, more passionate, and more sexual when delivered in this manner. It's as if you can't stop moving on top of your man and fucking the lights out of him.

As a result, the statement automatically transitions from soft-core to nearly hard-core.

But what if you say the same thing while looking at his crotch instead of his face? The statement's meaning abruptly shifts from a compliment to your lover to an expression of admiration for his manhood.

Similarly, the meaning of the same words varies depending on whether they are said during foreplay or while he is already buried deep inside you. In the former, it would read: "Your looks turn me on." In the latter case, "You're so hot." automatically translates to "You're so good in bed."

Dirty talk phrases with a vengeance:

Soft-core dirty talk appeals to our emotions, whereas hard-core dirty talk appeals to our animalistic natures. Women who do not use swearwords in everyday conversation may find it difficult to say words like "Fuck" and other profanities in bed. After all, if you despise swearwords, how can using vulgar language turn you or your partner on?

Consider the following: Swearwords irritate you, so you avoid using them. When you end up ejaculating these forbidden words in bed, it gives your lover the impression that you're losing control. Why? Because he's such a wonderful lover! Furthermore, the sex is so intense that there are no words in your good girl vocabulary to describe it.

I miss the taste of your cum on my tongue, for example.

I keep picturing you twirling your tongue around my clitter.

Make use of touch.

Combine steamy statements with enticing touches. Gently run your fingers along his inner arm, place your hand on his chest, or brush your fingers against his inner thigh.

Make up your secret codes.

Familiarity indeed makes a long-term relationship vulnerable. Having said that, you can also take advantage of this. The benefit of being together for a long time is that you know your man better than anyone else on the planet. In other words, you know exactly what makes the tip of his cock tingle. Create your lingo for lust. You can flirt in public and front of everyone's faces this way without anyone noticing. Admit it, this idea gives you an irresistible rush.

Ex: *I think it's about time we got our oil changed, don't you?*

The language of lust is unique to each individual. When they are exchanged between a husband and wife or two long-term lovers, they become an exclusive language. In this sense, dirty talk is

analogous to sharing an exciting secret with your lover. As a result, your relationship is strengthened.

CHAPTER 4:

GETTING YOUR LOVER IN THE MOOD FOR LUST

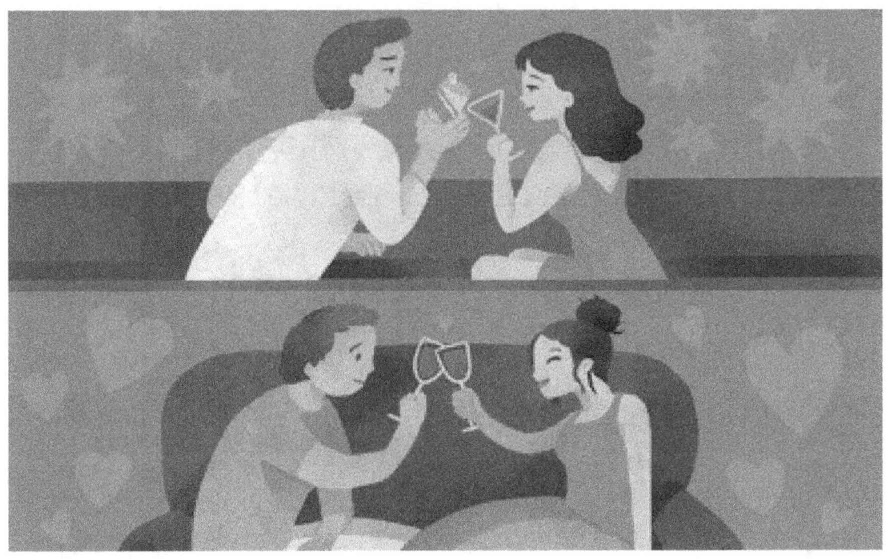

In this section, we'll look at the filthy, filthy things you can say to make your lover beg for sex.

What to Say to Her:

Women, as previously stated, associate romance with emotions. As a result, the quickest way to get between her legs is via her heart. To get her in the mood, show her that it's not just about sex with you.

In other words, you must demonstrate to her that you, too, have a sensitive side.

Surprise her with a lovely gift.

I've got a gift for you, whisper into her ear.

Then take her hand in yours and guide it to your crotch. Of course, she'll assume your not-so-surprising gift is your hard-rock penis. But what if you do keep a gift tucked away in there? Like a jewellery box or something else, she'll like. She's going to go weak at the knees. You'll have one grateful, enthusiastic partner in the sack.

Compliment her on her appearance and body.

Nothing in this world excites a woman more than the prospect of making love to a man who believes she is perfect.

I have to stop myself from coming in too soon when we're making love and I look at your face.

It takes my breath away when you're on top of me and those gorgeous tits bounce up and down.

You can bet she'll jump at any chance to show you that breathtaking view.

Recognize her previous efforts.

The more you appreciate your woman's efforts in bed, the more likely she is to do them again... and again.

Do you remember that strip dance you did? Even thinking about it gives me a hard-on.

Women like to believe that they are unique.

So, tell her that she's done something for you that no one else has ever done.

That was the best blow job I've ever had.

I had no idea a hand job could be so enjoyable!

Telling her she's the best at giving hand jobs/blowjobs will not only ensure repeat performances but will also inspire your woman to be more creative with her techniques. She'll want to live up to that reputation, after all.

Confidence piques the interest of women.

Men who know what they want and how to get it to turn them on. In other words, don't inquire. Inform her.

Don't say anything like, *"Can we have sex tonight?"*

Instead, say something like, "Tonight, I'm going to make you come as you've never come before."

While you're out in public, make her wet.

Stop staring at me like that, or I'll fuck you right here on the table. I don't care who is looking.

Things to Say to Him:

Sometimes all it takes is a promise to turn your man on.

I want to give you the best blowout you've ever had.

You could also tell your lover exactly what you want him to do to you.

I'd like you to lick my lips, neck, and breasts. Then I want you to kiss me from head to toe.

Make use of your hands.

I want you to kiss me... right here. (Place your hand between his and your legs.)

Remember that men enjoy feeling in control in the bedroom.

Tonight, I'll be your fuck doll. Consider all the things you want to do to me...

The key to building anticipation is to flirt with him in places and situations where he can't touch you.

Make a sexy promise to him before he leaves for work.

I wish we could spend the entire day in bed. We haven't done a 69 in a long time.

I'll be wearing that little French maid outfit you adore when you get home.

While he's at work, the image of you in that hot little number will be seared into his mind.

Alternatively, you can leave sexy suggestions in his pocket, such as a pair of handcuffs. When paired with such items, a simple note such as "For later." transforms into a dirty, super sexy phrase. When you're alone together, your lover will be bursting at the seams with all that pent-up passion.

Sticky notes can be placed in his underwear drawer, on his bathroom mirror, in his briefcase, or his lunch box. They don't have to be filthy all the time. They can be sweet with a subtle hint of eroticism at times.

Whisper something electrifyingly erotic into his ear when you're in a crowded place where he can't touch you.

I forgot to put on my pantyhose today.

I'm looking forward to our visitors leaving. When they do, I'm going to bind you to that chair and ride your cock all night.

Then proceed with your normal conversation.

When using obscene language to arouse your sexual soulmate, make sure you intend to follow through with your actions. Otherwise, you'll develop a reputation as an "all talk" lover. Your partner will become disoriented, confused, and tired of all the mixed signals you're sending. Worse yet, your words will lose their impact.

CHAPTER 5:

FILTHY WORDS FOR FOREPLAY

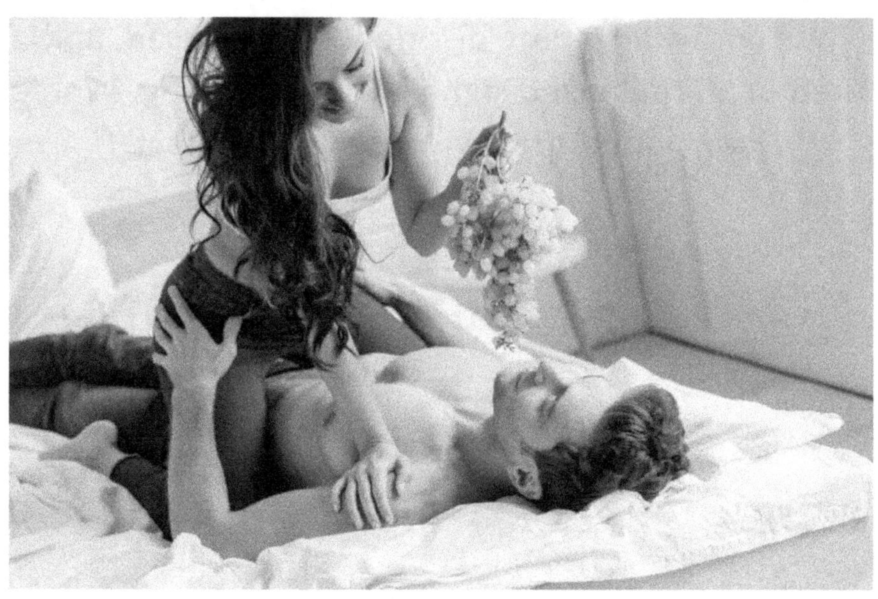

Finally, you find yourself behind closed doors. You've made all of those tantalizing promises. It's now time to deliver the goods!

What to Say to Her:

Use dirty talk during foreplay to make your lover feel safe and relaxed.

Simply relax. Allow your father to look after you.

Women are generally sensitive about their bodies, so make an effort to compliment whatever body part you're currently touching, kissing, or licking.

I enjoy burying my face in your breasts. They're so warm, soft, and lovely.

You taste like strawberries down there, baby.

Encourage your woman to take a more active role in foreplay by using bawdy talk.

I want you to put my cock in your sexy, filthy mouth.

Use foul language to reassure her that she's doing an excellent job.

Fuck! Your tongue feels fantastic on my balls. Don't give up, baby.

Use naughty language to express how much you've been looking forward to this moment.

Oh my God, I've been fantasizing about eating your cunt all day.

Use obscene language to describe what you've just done.

This is done to encourage a shy partner to be more vocal during foreplay.

For example, *I just tied you up and ripped your pants off.*

A statement like this prompts your lady to tell you what she wants you to do next.

Exude confidence when playing a role to become convincing.

She doesn't mind if you've got a beer belly. She'll believe you if you say you're a stud and mean it!

I'm your boss. You're a sex slave for me. Now, kneel and suck my cock. Things to Say to Him: Tell him how hot you think he is with naughty words.

Men, like women, enjoy knowing that they are desired.

My lady bits twitch a little when I touch your muscular arms.

Feed his ego. Make use of words that are appealing to his masculinity.

I like how broad your shoulders are. When you're on top of me, I feel tiny but safe and protected.

I enjoy the sensation of your chest hair against my breasts. They're so wealthy and manly.

Use vulgar language to describe what your lover is doing to you.

Ex: While he's fingering you, say something like,

"It feels so good when you slip your finger in and out of my hungry cunt." By the second, I'm getting wetter and wetter.

Yes, he's already doing it, but hearing the words come from your mouth will give him an extra, unexpected rush.

Do you like what he's doing? Use obnoxious language to let your man know he's on the right track.

Mmm... That's all. I like how you massage my breasts slowly and sensuously.

Don't agree with what he's doing? Use your foul language to divert his attention away from you.

For example, if he spends too much time sucking on one breast and it becomes raw, grab your other boob and say something like, "This baby's getting jealous."

Inform him of what you are about to do to him.

That brief moment in his mind when a fantasy is painted in his mind just before it becomes a reality is completely worth it.

I'm going to sit on your face now and let you eat me.

Make use of dirty talking to tell him what you want him to do next.

When you nibble on my clit, it feels so good. And my hot, wet pussy is hankering after your tongue.

This way, he'll know you want more and are prepared for him to stick his tongue out.

Because men are typically more aggressive in bed, when a woman asserts herself with confidence, it becomes a huge turn on for him.

You'll be begging me to take your cock in my hot, juicy cunt by the time I'm done playing with it.

CHAPTER 6:

DIRTY TALK WHILE DOING THE DEED

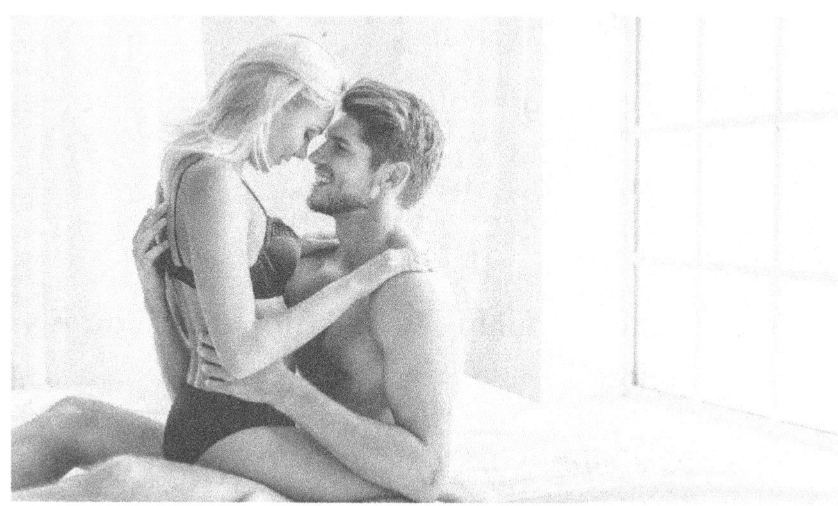

Things to Say to Her:

During intercourse, use dirty talk to make her feel safe, loved, and wanted.

Run your fingers through her hair while you're in the missionary position. Then, take a hold of her hair behind her head. Softly whisper into her ear as you thrust in and out.

Use dirty talk when you're in a position where you can make direct eye contact.

To convey sincerity, look deeply into her eyes.

Hold her close and whisper into her ear or against her neck if you're fucking her from behind. Touch her face and turn her head if possible so you can look into her eyes. Assure her that you love and respect her even if you treat her like a whore.

Ex:

You're my slut, my little slut. You are entirely mine, and I adore you.

I'm not sure I'll ever get tired of having sex with you.

If I could, I'd fuck you forever.

Describe the experience to her while you're deep inside her.

Of course, this includes telling her how nice it is to be in her pussy.

You're so fucking warm and tight. I wish I could stay here indefinitely.

Make her aware of the sexy things that are happening with her body.

See how drenched I've made you?

Hearing you pant like that... It makes me want to visit as soon as possible.

If she's on top, use foul language to motivate her.

Seeing you dominate me in this way... It's a total turn on!

Do you like what she's doing? Use obnoxious language to persuade her to continue.

That's it, baby, bounce that beautiful ass.

Use the repetition technique if you want her to keep doing something. This creates a trance-like state and taps into the subconscious.

You're a bad girl deep down, aren't you? You enjoy feeling my cock inside you, you filthy, filthy girl... You're so bad that I'm thinking about punishing you.

Tell her you're hers.

This cock is entirely yours.

Make it clear to her that she is yours.

*Woman, please knead. I'm going to f*** you from behind.*

Play with your breasts by putting your hands on them.

Extend your legs further. I want to take what is mine.

When issuing commands, use strong action words such as suck, lick, swallow, and so on.

Once you've mastered the art of giving orders, stack a series of commands to get her to do what you want.

You enjoy it when I fuck you **hard**. You're a naughty girl who enjoys a good time. You enjoy it when I push my cock so **hard** and rough.

After that, have your lover confirm this to you.

Tell me you like it tough.

69

If you're about to blow your wad on her, use your dirty mouth to warn her.

I'm going to fill your cunt with cum when I explode.

You're craving my cum, aren't you, dirty bitch?

What to Say to Him:

Let him know he's welcome as you let him in.

Oh, yes, I need you deep down inside.

Finally! All-day I've been thinking about your long, hard, throbbing cock.

Make his ego happy by letting him know how much of an impact he has on you.

Oh my God, my entire body is trembling.

Tell him how much fun you're having.

Don't dare to stop fucking me!

Describe the pleasurable sensations you're having in erotic detail.

It's so sensual the way your balls rub against my cunt.

Make him feel in command by using your filthy mouth.

I've been a terrible, terrible girl. Please punish me.

Use dirty talk to show him that you're not afraid to take it.

That's it, honey, fuck me so hard my cunt hurts.

Tell him you're his.

I am your whore. Make love to me as if I were your property.

I work as your sex slave. Take control of me.

I'm your plaything. Make use of me.

Use your lustful language skills to let him know you're ready to get rough.

Oh, pull my hair, baby!

That's it, honey, squeeze my tits even tighter.

Use dirty words to compliment his cock while he's deep inside you.

Oh, fill me up, baby!

Is your lover's pornographic speech making you uneasy? To cut it short, use your own filthy words.

Enough with the slander, Daddy. I'd rather you get your hands dirty on me.

CHAPTER 7:

GIVING MIND-BLOWING ORGASMS THROUGH DIRTY TALK

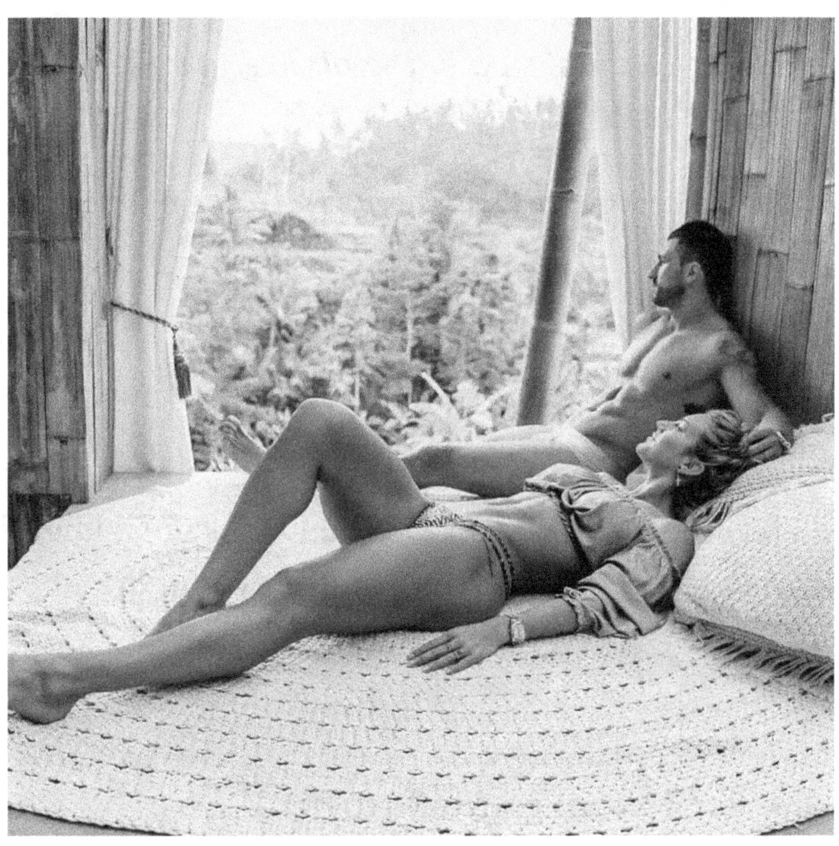

Things to Say to Her:

Playing on your woman's vanity is one way to bring her to the brink of a climax.

Tell her she's stunning. Let her know you think she's hot. Of course, in the dirtiest way possible.

I could come just by looking at your face, baby.

You are stunning. You fucking drive me insane.

When your ass is up in the air like this, it looks so hot. I can't stop fucking it up.

Do you realize how addictive the taste of your cunt is?

If there is one tip that is more effective than the previous one, it is this: Use filthy language to express your love for your woman.

I like the way you smell. When I fuck you like this, I love the way you moan. I adore everything about you...

Demonstrate your gratitude to her.

When she feels appreciated, she will relax, and the climax will be much easier to achieve.

Do you realize you're the best fuck I've ever had?

I wish I'd met you sooner. We were a perfect match.

Do you realize how thankful I am that your pussy is so tight? It's insane how good it feels.

Say her name aloud.

Incorporate her name into your passionate expressions of desire. This assures your woman that you are aware of who you are sleeping with. Furthermore, hearing her name from your lips makes the dirty talk feel more special and intimate.

Something about you, ____, brings out the animal in me.

Another way to get her to orgasm is to let her know you're almost at the climax.

Fuck, you're so hot I can hardly stand it.

I'm almost there, God. When I do this, I'm going to wash your filthy mouth with my cum.

Encourage her to express herself when she orgasms.

When you arrive, I can't wait to hear you moan.

You're going to call out my name when you arrive.

Finally, simply telling her to come will compel her to do so.

I'd like to have that juicy pussy squirt love juice all over my cock.

I want you to saturate my cock with cum.

I want your cum to be on these sheets.

Things to Say to Him:

Use filthy language to entice him to come.

Oh, honey, come get me.

I want to hear you scream my name when you come.

I'm after every last drop of your cum.

Use obscene language to alert him to the location where he can spill it.

Guys enjoy ejaculating all over you. It stems from their primal instinct to "mark their territory." Inform your man that you are permitting him to spill his sperm on your breasts, mouth, vagina, and so on. Knowing you're looking forward to his seed will make his release ten times more satisfying.

We're not going to stop until I can taste your cum in my mouth.

I'd like to have your cum all over my face.

I want your cum dripping down my leg when I wake up tomorrow.

Nothing can be more exciting for a man on his way to the top than knowing he's free to scatter his seed wherever he wants.

Tell me where you want to go.

I want you to pour it wherever you want when you come.

I'd like you to cover me in your cum.

The right words said at the right time can send your lover into an explosive, earth-shattering climax as he or she has never experienced before. Make sure you deliver these stimulating phrases throughout your partner's steady ascent to the pinnacle of pleasure. This can be accomplished by observing climactic signs such as rapid breathing, dilated pupils, and muscular contractions.

CHAPTER 8:

AMOROUS TALK AND AFTERPLAY

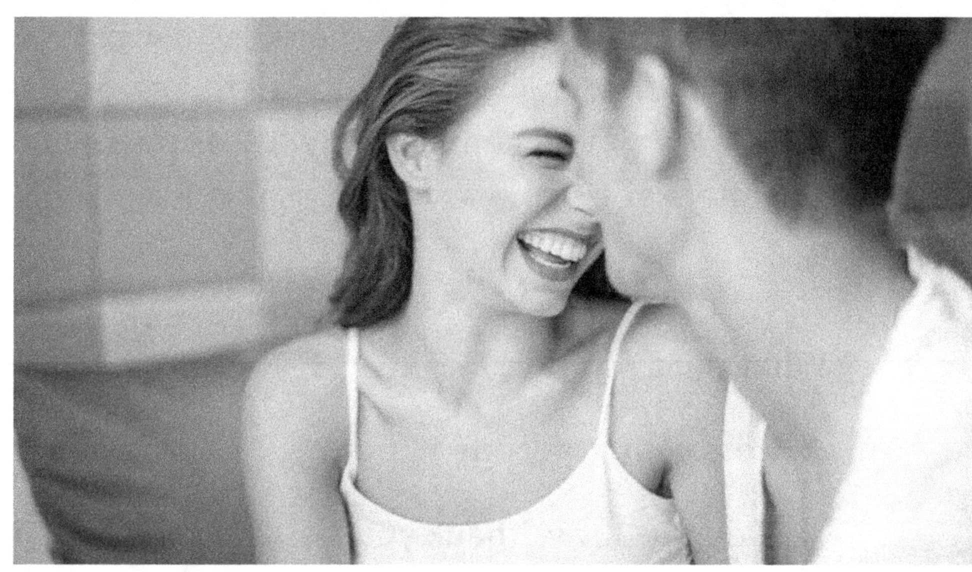

"Was it beneficial to you?"

Seriously? You can do much better than that. And you should.

People are more vulnerable after having sex. They've just given their all to their partners, and as they descend from the height of orgasm, they become especially vulnerable to judgment and rejection. They become aware of their naked bodies after being relieved of the animal lust that had consumed them. They begin to be concerned about their performance. They become concerned about whether or not their partner enjoyed the sex as much as they did. Reassure your lover before the anxiety sets in. Whether or not you're in love with your partner, you should have the decency to express your appreciation for him/her. That's not to say you should use the word "love" haphazardly. The first rule of dirty talk after sex is to be as honest as possible.

What to Say to Her:

Express your gratitude to her.

Don't just say "thank you," as if she's a prostitute who has just finished her services. Make her feel as if she's done something wonderful and special for you by using your skill in the language of love.

Do you realize how good you are in bed? I feel like a lucky jerk.

That was fantastic. I'm not sure what I did to deserve that.

I'm grateful to be here with you right now.

Compliment her body once more.

She's completely naked. She's not as horny as she used to be. She's thinking more clearly now, so she's starting to worry about how fat her ass might've looked while you were pumping her from behind. This is the part where you reassure her that everything is fine.

What was it that made me cum so hard? It was observing, grabbing, and slapping your round and perfect ass.

Remember the parts of the lovemaking that you enjoyed the most.

Then inform her of it.

The fact that you remembered it will both flatter and reassure her that she was fantastic in bed.

I noticed you licking my cum off your fingers... Damn. That completely blew my mind.

Women are naturally inquisitive, and some will not be able to resist asking you some follow-up questions.

They'll want to know if you had fun with the sex (even if it was pretty obvious because you were all over her face). If you've just slept with a girl for the first time, she's probably wondering if you'll call her again. When she asks you a question, just make sure you answer correctly.

For instance, when she asks, "Did you like it when I sucked your cock?"

Don't just say "yes" or mumble "uhuh." That's the same as saying her sucking... sucked.

Instead, tell her, "Yeah, I loved that part where you twirled your tongue around and around the tip of my cock while giving me a hand job." That was a fantastic movie.

Don't use dirty language to elicit compliments.

Of course, you want to know if it was beneficial to her. However, the goal of naughty talk after sex is to uplift your woman, not to feed your ego. Furthermore, begging for compliments makes you appear insecure and amateurish, which can be a turnoff.

Ex: Don't say things like, "Did you like it when I lifted your legs and filled you with my huge cock?" after sex.

Instead, say, "I admire your adaptability." I couldn't stop myself from laughing when I saw you with your legs raised like that.

Things to Say to Him:

Express your gratitude.

His ego is just as fragile after sex as yours. He'll have a million questions running through his head, such as how many times he forced you to come or if you came at all. Don't leave him in the dark. Inform him.

Your mouth is enchanted. Thank you very much.

Appealing to his masculinity is the most reassuring thing you can do.

You certainly know how to make a lady happy.

I like how you smell after you've had sex. It's very manly.

Use obscene language to persuade him to hold you after sex.

I wish we could sleep together while your cock is still inside me.

You can exaggerate slightly, but not significantly.

Don't say things like, "That was the most powerful orgasm I've ever experienced in my life."

After all, how many times can you possibly give your lover this compliment?

Instead, say something like, "You know, when you forced me to come, I felt a vibration all over my body." It was incredible.

He'll find out if you lie about having multiple orgasms right now. And then he'll start to wonder if he's been able to make you come all those times before.

CHAPTER 9:

STROKING YOUR LOVER'S EGO

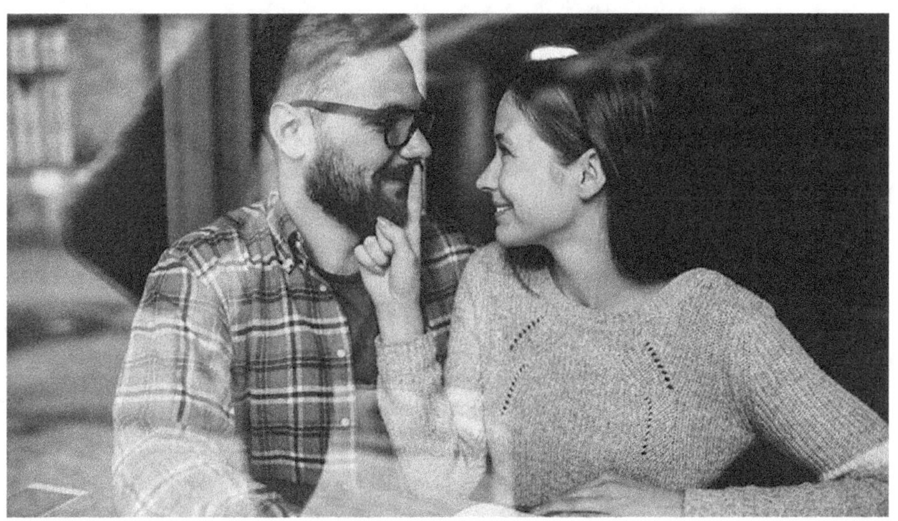

Why is it so critical to boosting your lover's self-esteem with words?

The simple answer is that the more attractive a person feels, the more likely he or she is to engage in sexual activity. Your wife/girlfriend may look like a supermodel, but if she hates what she sees in the mirror, you'll have a hard time convincing her that she can be a goddess in bed. It makes no difference if you get rock hard just by looking at her. If her subconscious mind believes she is undesirable, she will find it difficult to believe that anyone could lust after her. Furthermore, when a woman has a negative perception of her body image, she becomes apathetic or reluctant in bed. For example, she won't be open to trying out daring sex positions for fear of emphasizing her large thighs or belly. As a result, she ends up suppressing her most intense, wildest sexual fantasies.

The same is true for men. If a man looks in the mirror and sees an old, balding man with a potbelly, he'll have a hard time accepting the role of sex god. Instead, he'll end up playing the role of the slacker lover out of necessity. After all, that's what his body is designed for.

To be turned on for sex, one must first be turned on by his or her image. This means that one of the keys to having a great sex life is teaching your partner to love his or her own body. Use dirty talk to help your sexual soulmate realize his or her limitless lovemaking potential.

What to Say to Her:

Feed her compliments about her body and appearance regularly.

Don't just do it when you're having sex or pleading for some action between the sheets. The key is to tell her how sexy she is while you're in a non-sexy environment.

When she's bending over doing the dishes, tell her, *"I can't help but be distracted by your stunning rack."*

Congratulate her on her performance.

Cowgirl, you ride my cock like it's your birthright.

Women are often concerned about how they smell or taste down there. Assure her that everything is in order. She'll be less hesitant to have oral sex this way.

Your pussy tastes delicious. It's something I could eat all day.

Never compare her to your ex or any previous flings.

Even if you mean well, you can't get away with it.

Don't ever say things like, *"You give better blowjobs than my ex."*

Simply inform her that she provides excellent BJs. Period.

Things to Say to Him:

Men enjoy hearing that they are sexy as well.

Even if you're not in the mood to make love, tell him he's sexy.

I couldn't take my eyes off that bulge in your jeans. You're such a hottie.

Worship him and his cock.

Men regard their penises as extensions of their bodies. So, when you're on your knees performing fellatio, nuzzle your cheek against his junk and talk dirty to it.

My mouth longs for you. I can't wait to bring you inside. I can't wait to feel your cum pass down my throat.

Don't get too caught up in size.

Your compliments are easily misunderstood.

Don't say things like, *"I love it when you rub your little soldier up my ass."*

His brain will register the word "little," and he will interpret it to mean that his package is too small.

Also, don't refer to your lover's penis as a "giant cock" if you both know he's on the average side. A better option would be to express your gratitude for his iron-hard erection.

If you've been together for a long time, remind your partner of the days when you were wild and free, having sex whenever you could. Reminding your partner of his or her younger self can help rekindle his or her lust.

Ex: Him: Remember when we had sex in the sea? I came up behind you, pushed your bikini aside, and rammed my cock into you hard.

You were hot back then, and you're still hot now.

Her: Of course, I'll remember that. I had to lean back against your chest because my knees were so weak. Do you recall how many times you forced me to come that time? How about breaking that record today?

CHAPTER 10:

THE GUIDE TO STEAMY SEXTING

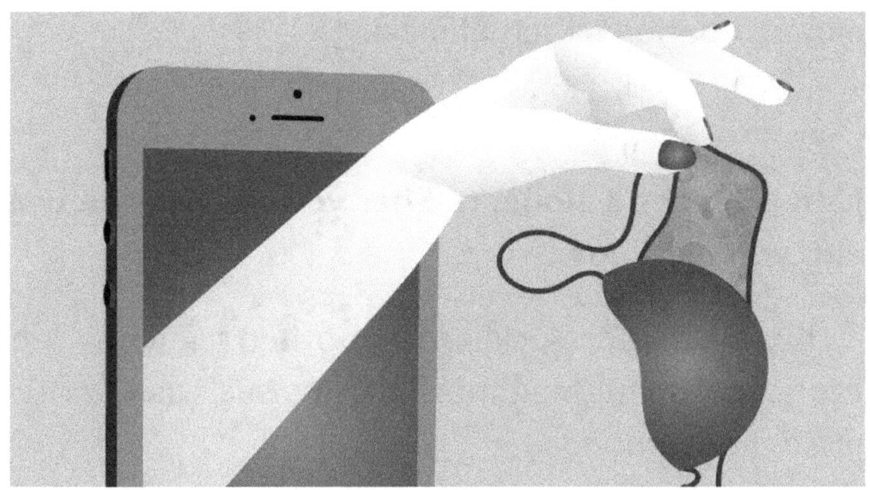

You've learned the majority of what you need to know about dirty talking by this point. Are you still unsure whether you'll be able to pull it off? Are you still unsure whether your partner is willing to engage in some titillating conversation? Sending sexy text messages to your lover is a great way to practice and test the waters.

What to Say to Her:

Inquire if she is alone.

When she's alone and doing nothing, it's the best time to start the sexy talk. This guarantees that you have her undivided attention. This also allows the dirty talk to progress to more obnoxious situations (as in masturbation or actual fucking).

If she says she's alone, tell her you to wish she was with you right now.

If you've been fucking each other regularly, feel free to say something more daring, such as *My cock misses you right now.*

You can begin with something gentler, such as I miss cuddling with you. I miss the smell of your hair... I'm kissing your neck...

No matter how mild your sexts are, always keep the physical stuff in mind.

Inquire as to what she is doing.

That is if you want to take things slowly. If she's up for sexting, she'll say something sexy like, "I'm about to take a shower." or "Nothing." "I was just folding my underwear."

Inquire as to what she is wearing.

If she's up for it, she might even lie about wearing granny panties and pretend to be wearing a black lacy thong.

Pose some provocative hypothetical questions.

If you're sexting with a girl you haven't had sex with yet, ask her questions like: If I were in your room right now, do you think we'd end up kissing?

What if everything goes wrong? What if you inadvertently offend the lady?

Then you should apologize. Sincerely.

A text message that says, "I'm sorry," *is a good example. I didn't mean to offend you in any way. I was just having fun. I'll be gentler.*

I swear. Xx

What to Say to Him:

Pose him some provocative hypothetical questions.

It's natural to be hesitant to start the dirty talk, but one way to pull it off and keep your ego intact is to start with ambiguous messages that may or may not allude to something sexual.

For example, *how would you keep me entertained if you were trapped in an elevator with me?*

What do you think we'd do if you weren't here and we were alone?

If you and your man have been fucking for a while, try a more titillating theoretical question: If I let you handcuff me and fuck me however you want, what would you do?

Use dirty sexts to let your lover know what to expect when you meet.

Tonight, I'm going to whip you until you pass out from pleasure.

Mixing the erotic with the mundane will astound him.

Do you mind if I stop by the grocery store later? We require garbage bags, fresh milk, olive oil, and so on. Oh, and don't forget about the whipped cream. I'm looking forward to licking it off your dick later.

Use sexy texts to surprise him with compliments.

Last night was a wild ride. I'll never forget how you drew me in with your tongue.

So, right now, I'm masturbating. I couldn't stop fantasizing about your cock.

Your cum is still lingering on my tongue.

Something about you makes me feel a little slutty. I secretly enjoy it.

Use dirty sexting to set the tone for your later-day lovemaking.

I'll be your Queen tonight. So brace yourself to get down on your knees and lick me until I tell you to stop.

You've been so good to me, baby. I've decided to let you fuck whichever hole you want when you get home.

Do you want to heighten his sexual anticipation? Respond to his questions with astonishment.

Ex: If he asks what you're doing, say something like, "I'm just playing with my pussy..." I'm missing you...

FINAL THOUGHTS

There is no such thing as the proper way to speak dirty. The definition of proper dirty talk is entirely subjective. Don't expect everything to go as planned. Even better, don't forget to laugh at any blunders you may make along the way. Remember that one of the keys to a great relationship is when couples can laugh with each other rather than at each other.

Perfect practice makes perfect. This applies to both sex and the art of dirty talking. The more you incorporate erotic phraseology into your sexy routine, the better you'll get. Don't, however, make the mistake of simply memorizing the examples in this book. Create your sexy lines. It's simple enough if you take a good look at your partner and consider what you like best about him/her. Try to be fully present the next time you put it on. Enjoy the sensation of her moist pussy flesh wrapping around your penis or his hard, muscular cock throbbing deep inside your vagina. Concentrate on the emotion, and the words will come to you. Do this with complete confidence that no one in the world knows and understands your lover's body better than you.

Be as natural as possible. Nothing kills mounting lust more effectively than an insincere compliment. Make an effort to be spontaneous rather than superfluous. Nobody expects you to recite a poem about his penis or deliver a powerful monologue about her vag. All your lover wants is for you to be yourself. Remember that the most important thing is to persuade your partner that you mean everything you say. So use the same words and expressions that you would. Don't say anything that might give your sexual soulmate the impression that he or she is having an affair with a stranger. Even if you're playing characters in your dirty dialogue, make sure you put some of yourself into it. This way, no matter how real things become, your lover's subconscious knows that he/she is still making love with you. You. In this world, the person he or she most loves, desires, and trusts.

Don't feel obligated to say things you don't want to say to please your partner. Your disgust will always betray you, no matter how good an actor/actress you are. Furthermore, keep in mind that you're investigating dirty talk not only for the pleasure of your lover but also for your own! So, sit down with your girlfriend/boyfriend or husband/wife and make your own rules while taking each other's fantasies and limitations into account. Finally, the best part about talking dirty with your lover is that it opens up new avenues for exploration. After all, what else can you do if you can talk like an expert seducer/seductress in bed? Talking dirty is only the beginning of revealing the deeper layers of your sexual persona. The confidence and liberation you gain from mastering the language of lust will inevitably lead you down the path to realizing your true carnal prowess, allowing you to become the best lover you can be.